Plantar Fasciitis Exercises and Home Treatment

Dr. George Best, D.C.

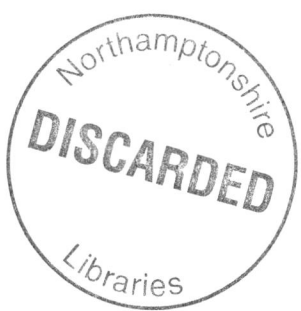

Plantar Fasciitis Exercises and Home Treatment

Copyright© 2014 George F. Best, D.C.

All Rights Reserved

ISBN-13: 978-1499691351

Table of Contents

Disclaimer and Additional Resources 1

Chapter 1: What Is Plantar Fasciitis? 2

Chapter 2: Exercises and Home Treatments 6

    Exercises 6

        Calf Stretching 7

        The "Toe Scrunch" 9

    Massage Techniques 10

        Foot Rolling 11

        Trigger Point Massage 12

        "Scraping" Massage Techniques 14

    Acupressure 18

    Using Cold and Heat 27

    Topical Analgesics 28

    Over The Counter Medications & Natural Remedies 28

    Laser Stimulation 31

    Shoes and Arch Supports 31

    Magnetic Therapy 32

    Energy Techniques 33

        Physical Energy Balancing Method 34

        Emotional Energy Balancing – Emotional Freedom Technique (EFT) 36

Chapter 3: Professional Treatment 42

Prescription Medication 42

Physical Therapy 42

    Ultrasound Therapy 43

    Iontophoresis 43

    Massage Therapy 43

    Taping 43

    Extracorporeal Shock Wave Therapy 44

Chiropractic / Osteopathic Manipulation 44

Acupuncture 45

Injections 45

Custom Fitted Orthotics 46

Rest 46

Night Bracing 47

Surgery 47

In Conclusion 48

Review and Connect 49

Disclaimer and Additional Resources

Every case is different and although the vast majority of plantar fasciitis sufferers will improve using the treatment methods presented, this book is not a substitute for professional evaluation and treatment. Some individuals may require different or additional treatments to the ones presented in this book. Readers are advised to pay close attention to the warnings and precautions that are included in this book and are advised to seek medical attention in the event that symptoms worsen or if new symptoms arise.

Although the author has tried to make the treatment instructions as easy to use as possible, certain methods may be somewhat difficult to understand from illustrations and text. For this reason, video instructions for some treatment methods, as well as means for contacting the author with questions, can be found on the author's website at:

www.AskDrBest.com/pfresources

Chapter 1: What Is Plantar Fasciitis?

Plantar fasciitis is a painful condition that involves irritation and/or degeneration of the plantar fascia, which is a tough, ligament-like tissue that runs along the bottom of the foot. The plantar fascia attaches at the heel bone and then fans out to attachments at the base of each toe and provides some of the support for the main arch of the foot. The plantar fascia is also important in walking or running, as it acts sort of like a spring as the foot propels you forward.

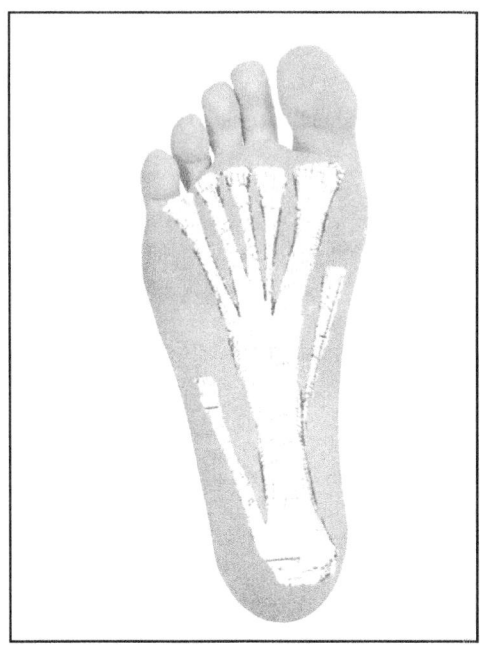

The Plantar Fascia

The symptoms of plantar fasciitis can occur pretty much anywhere along the bottom of the foot, but are most common around the heel, and it is common for plantar fasciitis to occur in conjunction with a heel spur. A heel spur (or calcaneal spur as it is also known) is an abnormal projection of bone that forms gradually on the bottom of the heel due to abnormal mechanical stress on the soft tissue attachments. Such spurs are often impressive to see on an X-ray and are naturally assumed to be a source of pain, but in fact the spurs themselves often produce no symptoms (despite how painful-looking they might be on an X-ray, many people with heel spurs don't feel them at all), with the associated pain coming from reactions in the soft tissues. With or without the presence of a heel spur, plantar fasciitis produces symptoms of sharp pain on weight bearing on the foot, usually worst after an extended period of sitting or lying down. Some people will also experience numbness, tingling, and/or swelling.

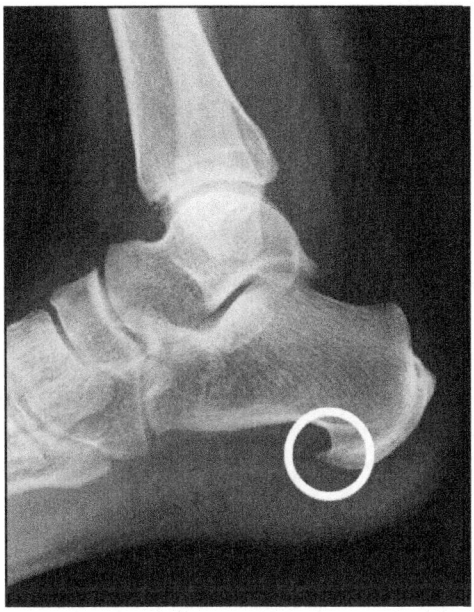

X-ray Showing a Heel Spur (Circled).

Although the –itis ending of the name would suggest that plantar fasciitis is an inflammatory condition, in the majority of cases there is little to no inflammation. While inflammation can occur with plantar fasciitis, it is more commonly a condition of structural breakdown and degeneration. It is believed to be brought on in most cases by repetitive micro-trauma – that is, minor damage occurring frequently over a long period of time. Distance running is so commonly associated with plantar fasciitis that the condition also goes by the common names of "jogger's heel" or "runner's heel", but it is certainly not exclusively a condition of runners. The condition frequently develops from repeated impact on the feet, following long periods of weight bearing (particularly on hard surfaces), and in people who tend to wear shoes without good arch support. Obesity is considered a risk factor (although plantar fasciitis commonly effects people who are not overweight), as is having flat feet.

There are a number of other conditions that are often confused with plantar fasciitis, including stress fractures, stone bruises, Morton's neuromas, peripheral neuropathies (degenerative nerve conditions such as from diabetes), and what doctors of chiropractic call "dropped metatarsal heads" (a misalignment of the joints at the base of the toes that produces pain in the ball of the foot). It can also occur in combination with other conditions and may be mistaken for a part of another pain syndrome. For example, sciatica will often cause pain that extends as far as the foot, and someone whose foot pain remains after other sciatica symptoms resolve might be assumed to still have sciatica when in fact they have plantar fasciitis.

To help distinguish it from other conditions, it is important to keep in mind the previously discussed symptoms and causative factors. For the sake of simplicity in self-diagnosis, there are two very common distinguishing features of plantar fasciitis. First, as mentioned previously, plantar fasciitis tends to be worst when weight bearing after prolonged rest, such as when you first get out of bed in the morning. The symptoms will then tend to improve somewhat after walking around a bit (the symptoms may gradually worsen with periods of prolonged walking or high-impact activities such as running, but the initial few minutes of walking after a period of extended rest tends to reduce symptoms). Most of the other conditions just mentioned will either be unchanged or tend to feel progressively worse with even short periods of walking. Although this reduction in symptoms with initial weight bearing activity can sometimes occur with sciatica, if there are sciatica symptoms in the foot they will almost always extend up the leg and not just be limited to the foot as is the case with plantar fasciitis.

The second distinguishing hallmark in most (but not all) cases of plantar fasciitis is tenderness along the medial (inside) front edge of the heel bone. Pressing firmly on this area will usually produce sharp pain which may extend along the plantar fascia towards the toes.

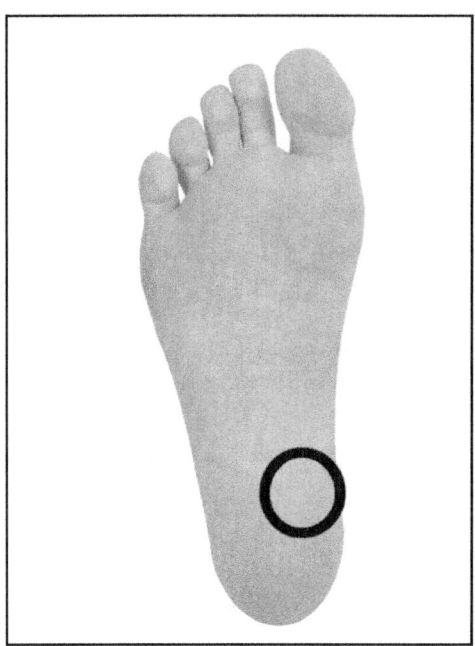

Plantar Fasciitis Diagnostic Hallmark: There will usually be a tender point on the front medial (inside) aspect of the heel bone in the area circled above.

If you have any doubt as to whether you might have some condition other than (or in addition to) plantar fasciitis, it is strongly advised that you be evaluated by a doctor to be sure not to neglect a potentially serious problem.

Chapter 2: Exercises and Home Treatments

<u>Exercises</u>

There are numerous exercises intended to help plantar fasciitis, but most of the variations accomplish basically the same thing: stretching the calf muscles. The reason stretching the calf is an almost universal recommendation for treating plantar fasciitis is that the calf muscles attach to the heel bone via the Achilles tendon. Tight calf muscles will pull the heel up and back, thereby placing abnormal tension on the plantar fascia and making it susceptible to injury.

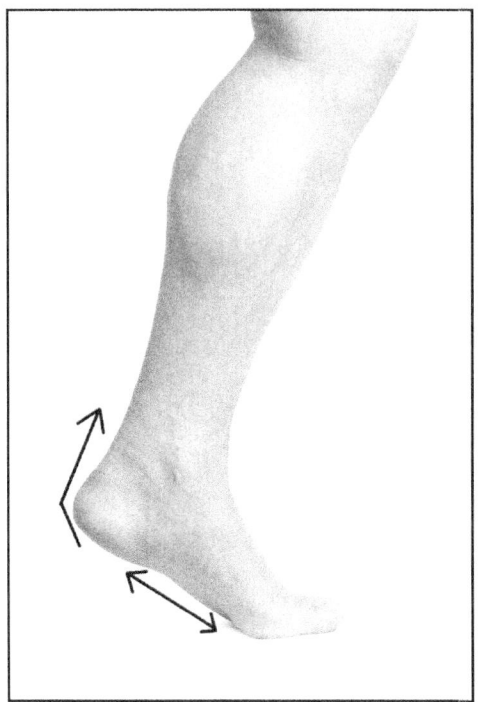

Tight Calf Muscles and Plantar Fasciitis: Tightness in the calf and Achilles tendon will pull the heel bone up and back, placing tension on the plantar fascia, resulting in abnormal wear and tear.

Calf Stretching

Since tightness in the calf muscles is an extremely common contributing factor in plantar fasciitis, calf stretches are pretty much a given when it comes to treatment. There are many different ways to stretch the calf muscles. A couple of simple methods are shown below. You don't really need to do more than one of the exercises. I suggest you choose the one that you like the best and that is the most convenient for you to do, and do it frequently.

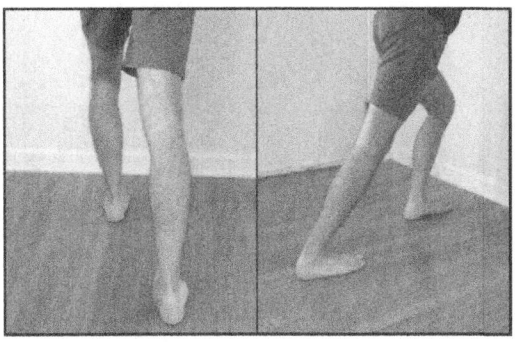

The Standing Calf Stretch (Two Views of the Same Exercise Shown Above): Stand near a wall you can place your hands on for balance. Place the foot of the leg to be stretched 1 to 2 feet behind the other leg, being careful to have the toes pointing straight ahead. Lean in towards the wall, bending the front leg while making sure to keep the back leg straight and the foot flat on the floor (don't allow the heel to come off the floor). You should feel a pull in the back of the calf on the back leg. For best results, hold the stretch for 15-30 seconds, switch legs (even if you only have symptoms on one side, it's best to stretch both), and repeat a few times on each leg.

For most people, the standing calf stretch is very effective and is convenient to do almost anywhere. Another option that can be done lying or sitting down is shown on the next page. Again, you don't really need to do both versions, just pick the one you prefer.

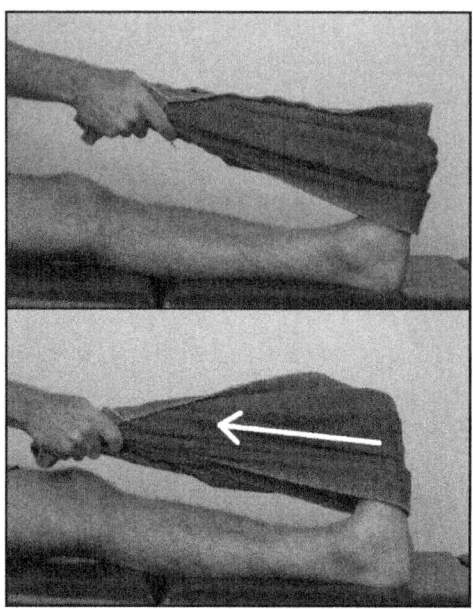

The Towel Calf Stretch: Lie on your back or sit with your leg straight on a flat surface. Loop a towel (a piece of rope or heavy therapy tubing can be used as well) around the ball of your foot and slowly pull your toes head-ward. Hold at the maximum stretch for 15 to 30 seconds, then switch legs and repeat a few times on each leg.

One commonly overlooked key to successful stretching is frequency, especially at first. While doing a few stretches once or twice per day might be sufficient to get good results, I recommend stretching a few times every hour you are awake (or as often as you can) for the first week, or until the symptoms go away. Once the calves have loosened up somewhat and the symptoms have decreased, you can reduce the frequency and then just stretch for a few minutes once or twice per day.

It is highly recommended that you then continue on this schedule as a lifetime preventive measure. Remember, exercises are forever, not just when you're having symptoms. If you started an exercise program to lose weight and then quit as soon as you reached your goal, you'd quickly start to gain back the weight you'd lost. Just like with exercise to get in shape, exercises used to treat a painful condition have to be continued to maintain the benefits. The things that caused the problem to develop in the first place are probably still a part of your life, so if you stop doing the exercises when the symptoms go away, chances are the symptoms are going to return.

The "Toe Scrunch"

The next exercise I suggest for both relieving plantar fasciitis and preventing it is the "Toe Scrunch". The toe scrunch is a strengthening exercise for the muscles at the bottom of the foot.

As was discussed in Chapter 1, one of the functions of the plantar fascia is to support the main longitudinal arches in the foot. The muscles provide the majority of arch support, so when the muscles are weak, there is more stress on the plantar fascia.

The toe scrunch is similar to grip exercises for the hands. Simply place a towel on the floor (a tile, wood, or other smooth flooring works best, as the towel will tend to cling to carpet), place your foot flat on the towel, and use your toes to scrunch it up.

Although it's a good idea to eventually make this part of your daily preventive exercise routine, take it slow when you first start with this exercise and only do it for 30 seconds to a minute at a time once or twice a day. If your foot muscles are very weak, you may find that the muscles get sore doing it every day, so you may need to do it every other day initially. Once you get used to it, you can increase the time somewhat to one or two minutes at a time once or twice per day.

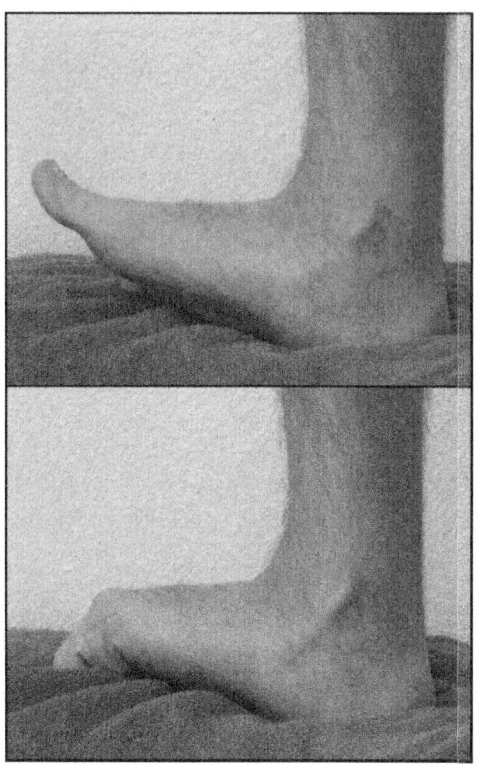

The Toe Scrunch Exercise. Place a towel on the floor, then place your foot on the towel and curl your toes to "scrunch" the towel up beneath them. Uncurl your toes, raise your foot slightly, then set your toes on the towel and curl them again. Work the towel with your foot for a minute or so at a time, or until the muscles feel tired. If you overdo, your foot may get sore or begin to cramp, so take it easy at first.

Massage Techniques

Massage can be very helpful for alleviating plantar fasciitis. While I do recommend professional massage therapy when possible, it is good to use self-massage as well.

Foot Rolling

One commonly-recommended method of self-massage for plantar fasciitis is rolling the foot on a golf ball, bottle, or other firm, round object. Of course, there are also foot massage devices available for this purpose, but make-shift rollers work just fine and there's not really a need to spend a lot of money on a special foot roller. I believe that a spherical object such as a golf ball is generally more effective than a cylindrical object in order to be able to work the foot at multiple angles. On the other hand, it's also better to do the treatment than to put it off indefinitely until you remember to get a package of golf balls, so my recommendation is to go ahead and get started using whatever you have. A tennis or racquet ball (not ideal because they are a little too soft), a baseball, a length of metal or plastic pipe, a cylindrical thermos bottle, or even a ball of twine or a roll of tape could potentially be used for this purpose.

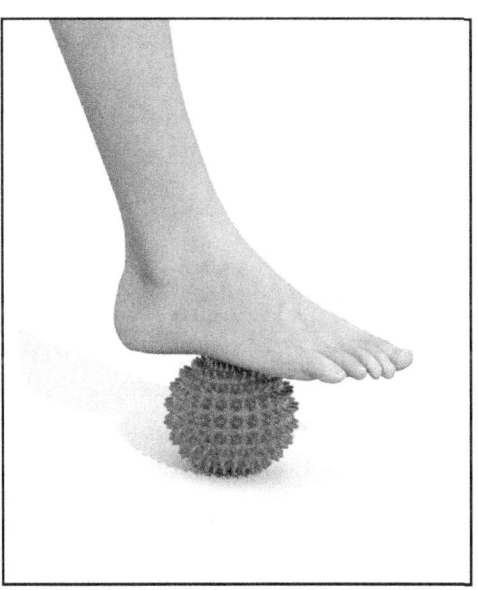

There are devices specifically made for foot rolling, such as the massage ball shown above. Special equipment is not necessary though and a golf ball, baseball, bottle, or piece of pipe will do the job.

While the rolling itself is the most important thing, some people get additional benefit by adding heat or cold to the equation (some experimentation is required to see if one or the other is helpful for you). For example, to apply heat, one option is to sit on the side of a bath tub (or an actual hot tub if you have one available) and roll the foot on a waterproof roller of some sort (a golf ball works very well for this) in warm water. For cold, a frozen bottle of water (use a plastic bottle – glass will often crack and explode in the freezer!) works well – just be sure to wear a sock to prevent excessive cooling of the skin and frostbite.

In any case, you want to roll the foot using moderate pressure – enough that you feel some tenderness initially, but not so much pain that you are gritting your teeth to get through it. A few minutes of rolling at a time up to every few hours each day is ideal during the initial stages of treatment, but if circumstances don't allow such a frequency, just do it as often as you can.

I have one other tip about foot rolling that I'm a little hesitant to add out of fear of someone being offended, but it does work, and although the story behind it is a bit risqué, I think most people will find it amusing. One of my patients told me that she had used a "personal massager" as her roller. She reported that the vibration combined with the rolling was quite soothing and did a much better job of easing her symptoms than the golf ball did. She added that it also worked better than her husband – at massaging her foot, as she clarified with a laugh!

Trigger Point Massage

This brings me to trigger point massage. Rolling the foot will usually work most of the tight knots of soft tissue contraction, but seeking out those points with your fingers and then massaging them with deep finger tip pressure or a massager of some kind will sometimes get to some of the most symptomatic spots that may get missed with foot rolling. The angle of pressure can make a huge difference in the sensitivity of a given spot, so actually checking with your hands is definitely worth the extra effort.

Once a tender point / trigger point (the distinction is that a tender point is only locally tender, whereas a trigger point may produce referred pain some distance from the point of pressure) is found, then you can apply deep pressure to it for 10 to 30 seconds and repeat as necessary until the tenderness and any referral pain dissipates.

If you have relatively strong fingers, you can just use your hands to apply the pressure, but you can also use a massage tool of some sort. While there are such tools specially made for massage, you can easily improvise one as well. For example, the handle of a screwdriver or other hand tool works quite well for this purpose. Here too, an electric vibrating massager can be helpful, either to apply pressure on the tender/trigger point or as a more general massage for the foot to get the circulation moving (and reduce sensitivity) before proceeding to the deep pressure massage.

Before beginning with these methods, it's important to define what "deep pressure" is, especially if you are using some type of tool other than your fingers to do the massage. For the treatment to be effective, you're usually going to need to use enough pressure that there will be some discomfort while working on the points. Some points will be much more sensitive than others and some people have a much higher pain tolerance than others. While some pain is usually necessary to achieve the gain, it's not advisable to subject yourself to excruciating pain, as being too aggressive with the massage is likely to make your foot even more sore than it was to begin with and can potentially damage the tissue. It's far better to "ease into things" and do less intense massage on a more frequent basis initially than to try to work everything out at once. As a general rule, I recommend starting out by applying about 10 to 15 pounds of pressure on the points.

So, how do you know when you're applying 10 to 15 pounds of pressure? If you have a bathroom scale, you can push down on it with your fingers/thumb/or whatever massage tool you may be using to get a feel for that amount of pressure.

Another trick is to use a gallon bottle of water or milk (make sure the cap is on tight!) and rest it cap-down on your hand, then mimic that amount of pressure with your fingers/thumb/massage tool. Since a gallon weighs approximately eight pounds, you can apply a bit more pressure than the bottle, but it will help you get an approximation of how hard to press.

After you've done it a few times and have an idea of how your body is going to react to the treatment, you can step up the pressure somewhat if you want to, but you don't need to cause yourself undue pain to get results.

Now that you know how hard to push, you need to know where. Common locations to look for tender/trigger points in need of massage are shown in the illustration on the next page.

14 • Plantar Fasciitis Exercises and Home Treatment

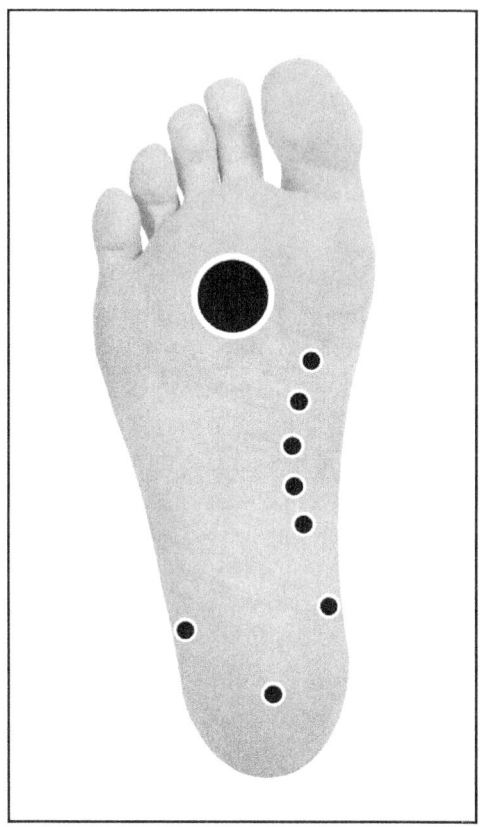

Trigger Point Massage – Common locations for points in the foot are shown above. Use firm fingertip or thumb pressure to locate areas of contraction/tenderness. Apply firm pressure with your fingers or an assistive tool for 10 to 30 Seconds at a time and repeat as necessary until the tenderness and any referral pain (pain that spreads out from the point of pressure) dissipates.

The large area in the ball of the foot can also be smacked 20-30 times with your fist to stimulate circulation and ease plantar fascia tension.

"Scraping" Massage Techniques

Some techniques such as Graston and ASTYM use a "scraping" type of massage using various tools to alleviate areas of constriction in the soft tissue. These methods can be quite effective, especially in cases of plantar fasciitis related to trauma or overuse injuries where there has been scar tissue formation. The drawback of these methods is that they can be quite painful and, if done too aggressively, they can actually make things worse. For this reason, as with the trigger point / tender point massage, I recommend you take things slowly.

There are a lot of common household objects that can be used for scraping massage. Pretty much anything that has a smooth surface without any sharp edges can be used. I suggest using an ordinary stick pen that is uniform in diameter along its length. A pen is usually just long enough to allow you to hold onto the ends and cover the width of the tissue that needs to be scraped, plus it automatically limits the amount of leverage you'll have so there's little chance of pressing in too hard and causing injury.

If you've had Graston, ASTYM, or some similar technique from a professional therapist before, you know that they tend to apply quite a bit of pressure and you may find that using a pen as your massage tool doesn't allow you enough leverage to match what you may have experienced with your therapist. That's to be expected and it is my intent that you NOT be able to perform quite as intense of a therapy on yourself. Bear in mind that professionals who use these techniques have undergone extensive training in how to use them safely. You have not had such training and getting some instructions from a book or even a video is simply insufficient for you to be able to safely apply a highly intense treatment modality. To avoid injuring yourself, I strongly recommend you stick to the less-intense methods that are discussed here.

Finally, while those with relatively mild plantar fasciitis can usually tolerate trigger point and scraping massage every day, in more severe cases, this may be too much. When starting out, I recommend these methods be used every other day until you have done them a few times and have a good idea of how your body will respond. If you don't have any major issues with post-treatment soreness after the first few sessions, but you haven't quite been able to eliminate your symptoms, you can try increasing the massage techniques to daily if you wish.

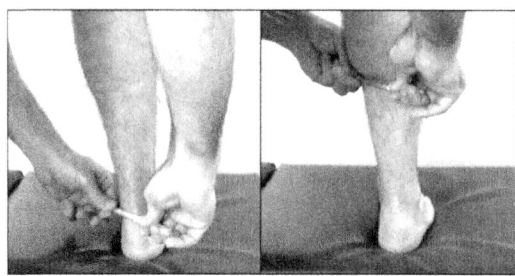

Scraping Massage of the Calf Step 1: First apply some lotion to your lower calf to allow the scraping tool (in this case, a ball point pen) to slide easily over the skin. Start at the bottom of the Achilles tendon just above the heel bone and slowly slide up the inner edge of the tendon with firm pressure until you reach the bottom of the "meaty" part of the calf. Repeat 6 to 8 times before shifting the tool so that it is directly over the middle of the Achilles tendon.

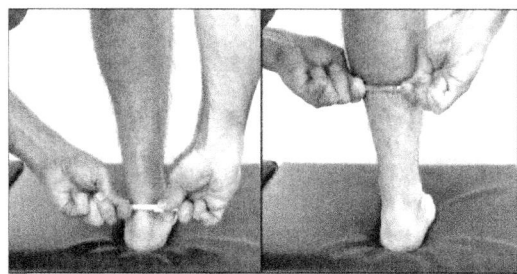

Step 2: Again, start at the top of the heel bone and slowly slide upwards to the bottom of the calf muscle with firm pressure. Repeat 6 to 8 times before shifting the tool over to the outer edge of the tendon.

Plantar Fasciitis Exercises and Home Treatment • 17

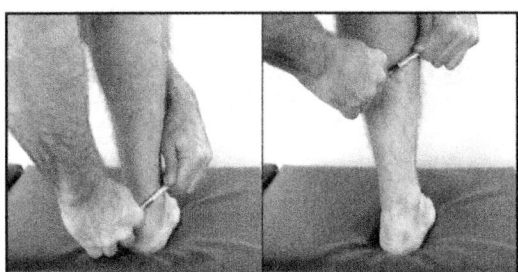

Step 3: You may need to angle your tool slightly to get around the lateral malleolus (the "bump" on the outside of the ankle). Slide up the outside edge of the Achilles tendon with firm pressure to the calf muscle as before and repeat 6 to 8 times.

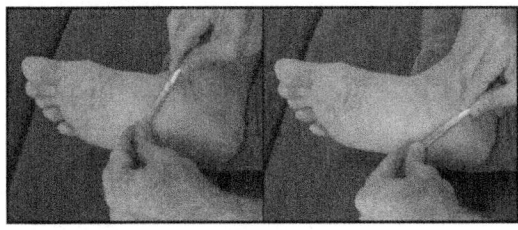

Scraping Massage of the Plantar Fascia Step 1: First, apply lotion to the bottom of your foot, and rub firmly and briskly up and down the foot to get the circulation moving and get things loosened up a bit. Start on the back part of the medial arch (in the fleshy area behind the bony projection in the middle of the arch). Press in with firm pressure and slowly slide the massage tool back towards the edge of the heel. Repeat 6 to 8 times.

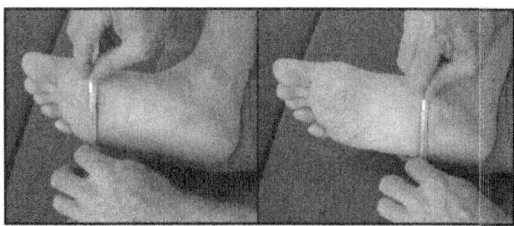

Step 2: Move the tool to cover the width of the foot, just behind the big toe pad. Press in firmly and slowly move the massage tool towards the front edge of the heel bone. Repeat 6 to 8 times.

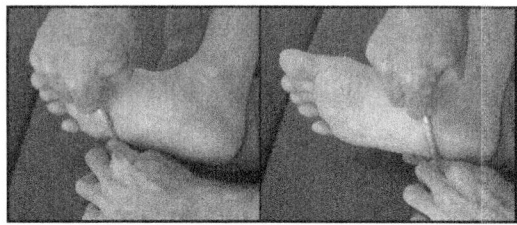

Step 3: Finally, move the tool to the outer edge of the bottom of the foot, begin behind the ball of the foot and press in and slide the tool along the outside of the sole of the foot to the edge of the heel bone. Repeat 6 to 8 times.

Acupressure

Although similar to tender/trigger point massage in terms of technique, acupressure is done with a different intent. Massage is intended to directly affect the tissue being worked on by means of mechanically loosening restrictions and increasing circulation and lymphatic flow. Acupressure is intended to change the flow of energy through what are known in traditional Asian medicine as meridians.

Meridians and energy flow are concepts that are still pretty unfamiliar to most Westerners. In very simple terms, meridians are a means of "wireless" communication in the body like using a cell phone, whereas nerves provide a "wired" communication system like a "landline" telephone. Both the meridian system and the nervous system are very important and used by the body to assess conditions and coordinate the body's response to its environment. Acupressure uses meridian points to alter the balance of energy flow through the body and thereby can affect a variety of body processes, including things like pain and inflammation. Because acupressure is dealing with energy balance, it is often applied on points that, from an anatomical perspective, might seem to have nothing to do with the area or complaint being treated. For example, as you'll see in the points that follow for treating plantar fasciitis, some of the points to be stimulated lie quite some distance up the leg from the foot, and one point is even on the palm of the hand - about as far away from the foot as you can get!

One other thing to be aware of is that most meridians are named according to associations with the energy flow of certain organs, such as the gallbladder meridian, the heart meridian, the stomach meridian, etc.. You can think of these organ names for the meridians more like radio stations named for the organs rather than being the organs themselves. For example, someone who has had his or her gallbladder removed still has a gallbladder meridian. Ultimately, the name of a given meridian point is primarily for reference, not to indicate that your symptoms are due to some type of organ problem.

Acupressure points can be stimulated in a number of ways and there's not really one way that's universally better than another, so it's really just a matter of personal preference. I suggest trying a few different methods and using the one or ones you find easiest to do and most effective. So, before I go into what acupressure points to treat, let's first discuss the various options for treating them.

The first method is, as the name acupressure suggests, to simply apply pressure. This will be similar to how the trigger point therapy was applied. You can either apply constant pressure for 30 to 60 seconds per point, or you may find it more effective to "pulse" the pressure – alternating pressing in and releasing every second or so. Pulsing can also be done using a "clickable" ball point pen with the button on the end of it. Basically, just place the button on the point and repeatedly push in (not far enough to actually "click" the pen as this will slow the pulsing down too much) and release as rapidly as possible. Another option is to tap on the points with a fingertip, again for 30 to 60 seconds per point. Each point can be stimulated repeatedly throughout the day. As a general rule, any points that are tender to pressure can benefit from additional stimulation. If you are limited on time, I suggest focusing on stimulating only the most sensitive points.

One other method that is somewhat faster and easier for many people and works quite well in most cases is to stimulate the points with a laser pointer (available in most office supply stores). For best results, I recommend using a red laser in the 630-635 nm wavelength range (avoid green lasers as they generally don't work very well for this purpose). Simply shine the laser on the point for about 10 to 30 seconds per point. For best accuracy, I suggest you actually touch the laser wand to the points.

Now that we've covered how to stimulate the points, I'll go over what points to stimulate and where to find them in the images that follow. Some of the points can be a little difficult to find at first even using the pictures as a guide. In many cases, the points will be somewhat tender or produce a tingling or aching sensation when you press on them and that's a good indicator that you are on the right spot.

If there's no tenderness or unusual sensation and you're not sure if you're exactly in the right place, don't worry about it too much – there will be some effect from the stimulation even if you're not exactly on the point. Generally it's best to stimulate the points on the side of symptoms, but there's no harm in stimulating the points on both sides if you like and it may provide additional benefits in some cases.

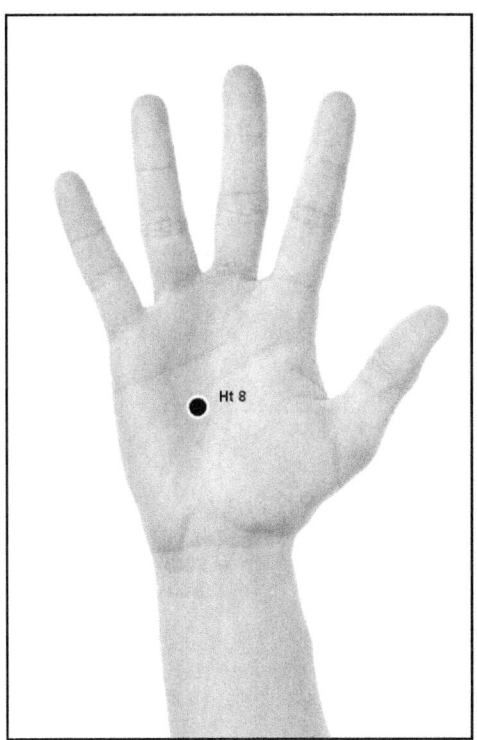

Ht (Heart) 8: Found in the palm of the hand on a line down from the ring finger to where it meets a line across the hand from the web of the thumb.

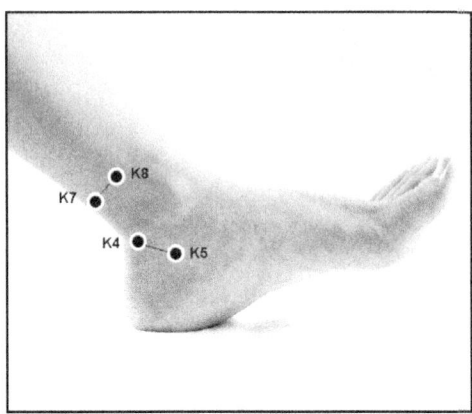

Kidney Meridian (K) Point Pairs for Plantar Fasciitis: The points shown above work best when stimulated simultaneously in pairs (indicated by the line joining the points).

K7 is located at the front edge of the Achilles tendon on a line just above the top of the medial malleolus (the bony "bump" on the side of the ankle). K8 is just forward of K7 on the back edge of the tibia bone.

K4 is in the depression behind and below the medial malleolus. K5 is found about 1 finger width below and in line with the back edge of the medial malleolus on a small bony projection.

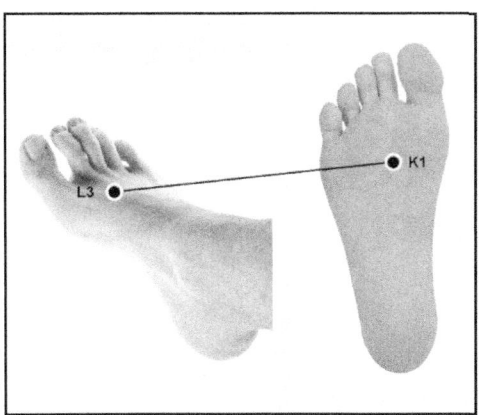

Liver (L) and Kidney (K) Pair: These points should also be stimulated at the same time, which can be done with one hand "pinching" the top and bottom of the foot.

L3 is located on the top of the foot in the groove where the first and second metatarsal bones meet (follow the space between the first and second toe until the bones come together). K1 is on the bottom of the foot in the depression (easiest to see if you curl your toes under) found on a line drawn from between the base of the second and third toe to the center of the heel alongside the metatarsal pad of the big toe.

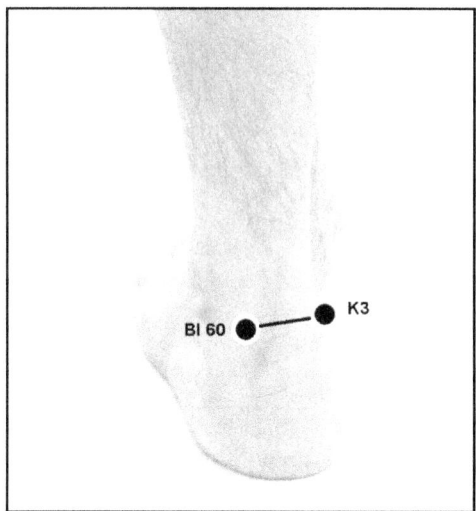

Bladder (Bl) and Kidney Pair (K): This pair of points should be stimulated simultaneously and is particularly useful in cases where there is a heel spur present. Bl 60 is located in a depression on the outside (little toe side) edge of the Achilles tendon just above the heel bone. K3 is in the depression on the inside (big toe side) edge of the Achilles tendon just above the heel bone.

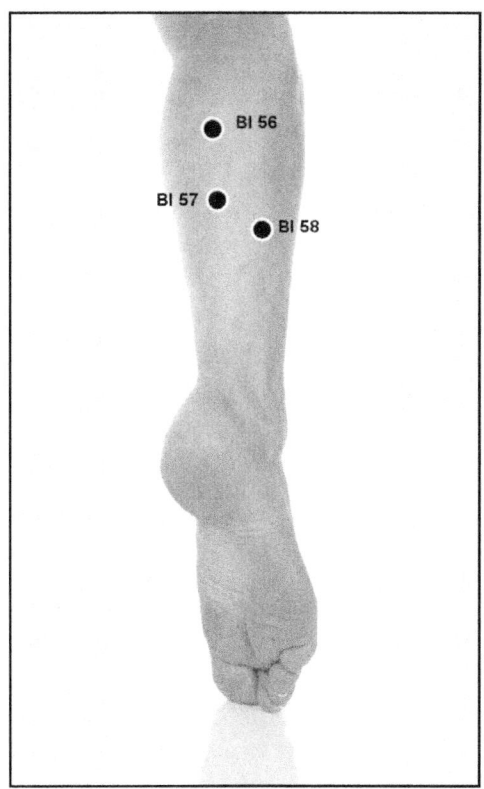

Other Bladder (Bl) Meridian Points for Plantar Fasciitis: Bl 56 is located in the center of the belly (the "meaty part") of the calf muscle. Bl 57 is found in the center of the depression at the base of the belly of the calf muscle and is easiest to locate if you stand on your "tip-toes". Bl 58 is located on the back edge of the fibula bone about 1 finger width to the side and below Bl 57.

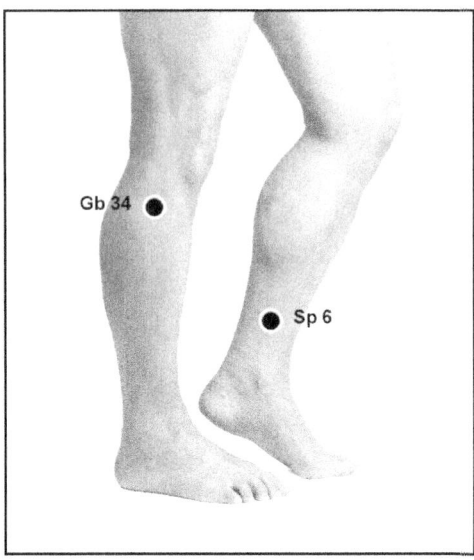

*Gallbladder (Gb) and Spleen (Sp) Points: Gb 34 is located in a depression in front of and just below the head of the fibula (which will be the bony bump on the outside of the leg just below the knee). Sp 6 is located on the back edge of the tibia bone approximately 3 finger widths above the top of the medial malleolus (the big bump on the big toe side of the ankle). *Note the picture shows Gb 34 on the right leg and Sp 6 on the left leg. It is recommended that the points be stimulated on the side of symptoms.*

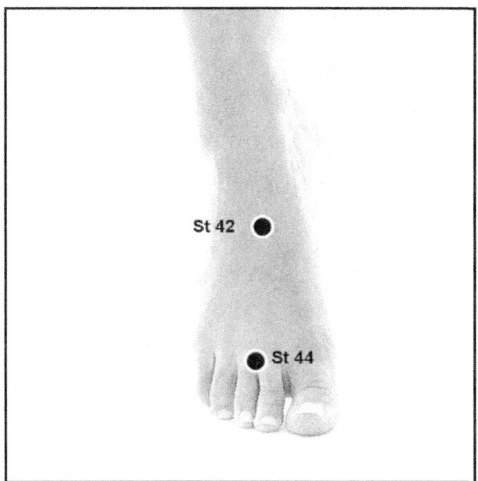

Stomach (St) Meridian Points for Plantar Fasciitis: St 42 is located in the top of the depression between the big toe tendon and the junction of the tendons going to the other toes (easiest to find if you use your foot muscles to dorsiflex your toes –that is, point them up toward your head). St 44 is in a small depression on top of the foot just behind the web of the second and third toes.

Using Cold and Heat

We briefly discussed cold and heat when we talked about rolling massage. Plantar fasciitis varies considerably from one case to the next with regards to the response to cold and heat, so it's a good idea to try both and see which works best for you. Some people like to alternate cold and heat. I have not found this to be superior in results to just using the one the works the best, but there's no harm in alternating them if this is your preference.

Cold can be applied by means of the frozen water bottle as already discussed, or with a soft ice pack. Gel packs are excellent for this as they will conform to the surface of the foot. Another option is to use a package of frozen peas or corn nibblets. Regardless of what you use, it's recommended that you use a thin sock or otherwise separate the cold pack from the skin to avoid causing frost bite. Apply the cold pack for about 10 minutes starting from when you begin to feel the cold through the cloth layer.

There are various options for applying heat, from soaking the foot in a warm bath tub, to using a chemical heat pack, to using a heating pad. If you do use a heating pad, it's best to get one with a moist heat insert to avoid dehydration of the tissue. Another make-shift option is to put a damp towel in a microwave oven and heat it up (carefully check the temperature to make sure it's not so hot that it will burn you). For heat, apply for about 10 minutes at a time.

Whether you use ice or heat, they can be applied up to every two hours or so, or at least until the skin has returned to normal temperature. If you are alternating cold and heat, the combination can be applied up to every two hours.

Topical Analgesics

There's a wide variety of products that can be used topically to temporarily reduce symptoms. While some may contain aspirin or some other anti-inflammatory agent, most only relieve symptoms by means of neurological distraction. Basically, whether the products are cool feeling, hot/burning feeling, or some mixture of the two, they stimulate nerves that block the conscious part of the brain from feeling the pain. There's nothing wrong with using these products for temporary pain relief, but be very careful when using them with cold packs, especially cooling products such as those containing menthol. A cold pack applied over an area that has been treated with Icy-Hot, Biofreeze, or a similar product can quickly cause frostbite damage to the skin before you feel it. So, if you're using topical analgesics, be sure they've completely worn off or thoroughly wash them off before applying a cold pack.

Over The Counter Medications & Natural Remedies

Over the counter medications may be helpful in some cases of plantar fasciitis and not at all in others. The most popular products are the Non Steroidal Anti-Inflammatory Drugs (NSAIDS) which include aspirin, ibuprofen, and naproxen as the top-sellers in the OTC market. Pain relievers containing acetaminophen (which does not have any anti-inflammatory effect) are also popular. I have not seen any of these products to be particularly effective for plantar fasciitis, but they may provide a small degree of pain relief on a temporary basis. I do not recommend such products for daily long-term use though as they do have the potential to cause liver and kidney damage. Furthermore, there is evidence that NSAIDs inhibit the body's ability to produce collagen and therefore likely accelerate the progression of degenerative joint and soft tissue conditions (such as plantar fasciitis).

There are numerous nutritional supplements, herbal products, and homeopathic remedies being promoted for the treatment of pain and inflammatory conditions.

The list of possible supplements and remedies is incredibly long, so for the purposes of simplicity, the following recommendations has been limited to readily available supplements and remedies that have some amount of validation from scientific research and/or strong anecdotal evidence supporting their effectiveness and safety.

The suggestions that follow are in regards to particular vitamins, minerals, herbs, etc., not to particular brands. With regards to brand-name products, you should be aware that marketing hype often far exceeds actual results that can be expected with a given product. Due to variability in the availability of certain products in different parts of the world, I do not make specific recommendations regarding brands. When it comes to choosing a brand, whenever possible, my recommendation is to look for a product that uses independent lab certification of the potency and purity. Optionally, it may be helpful to research the product on Amazon.com or other shopping websites to look at user reviews of the product.

The first group of potentially helpful supplements are those that inhibit the inflammatory response and thereby reduce swelling and pain. Although most cases of plantar fasciitis are not inflammatory in nature, there does still seem to be a therapeutic effect with both pharmaceutical and natural anti-inflammatories, presumably because these products also tend to have a separate analgesic effect. There are many anti-inflammatory supplements, but among the most popular and best-documented by scientific research are: omega-3 fatty acids (EPA and DHA – from fish oil, krill oil, walnut oil, or flax seed oil), bromelain, hesperidin, quercetin, curcumin (turmeric), MSM, ginger, and aloe vera.

Different ones work to varying degrees for different individuals, but from my experience, I would say that omega-3 fatty acids and turmeric/curcumin, are among the most effective with the least tendency to cause gastrointestinal upset. Both also have additional documented health benefits, so even if they do not help with plantar fasciitis symptoms, they are probably worthwhile from a general health perspective. Dosage recommendations vary widely, but my suggested starting dosages are: 1000 mg of omega-3 fatty acids with meals once to twice per day and turmeric/curcumin containing 200 to 300 mg of curcuminoids taken once to twice per day with food.

***CAUTION: If you are already taking either over-the-counter or prescription anti-inflammatories, or you are on blood-thinning drugs such as Coumadin (Warfarin), it is strongly recommended that you consult with a pharmacist or licensed healthcare provider before starting any nutritional anti-inflammatories as there is a potential for dangerous interactions.

Homeopathic remedies for reducing pain and inflammation may also be useful, and there are many such remedies. Although the findings of formal research studies have been mixed, it has been my observation that homeopathic Arnica (either taken orally and/or gel/cream applied topically) works quite well for many people. For best results with homeopathy, I recommend consulting with a homeopathic physician to be formally evaluated to determine the remedy that is best suited to your particular needs.

Although not a cause of actual plantar fasciitis per se, one common nutrient deficiency that can produce foot and leg cramping and pain is potassium deficiency. Potassium deficiency is most commonly seen in individuals who lose a lot of fluid through perspiration, vomiting, or diarrhea, and in people with kidney disease. It can also occur as a side-effect of certain medications, such as those for high blood pressure – especially diuretics. Mild potassium deficiency can usually be corrected safely by simply getting more potassium in the diet. Although bananas are the classic high-potassium food, many other foods are as good or better sources of potassium. These include melons, avocados, oranges, most green leafy vegetables, and black-strap molasses. Potassium supplements are also available, but before taking high doses of potassium supplements, it is strongly recommended that blood testing be performed to measure potassium levels – too much potassium can be dangerous!

One other deficiency that commonly produces foot pain, although usually as a part of all-over body pain, is Coenzyme Q-10 (or CoQ10 for short). This deficiency is frequently the result of a side-effect of cholesterol-lowering drugs. There are two options in handling the deficiency. The first is to supplement with coenzyme Q-10 at a suggested starting dose of 200 mg per day. If this relieves symptoms, the dosage can usually be reduced to 50 to 100 mg per day for maintenance. If there is no benefit, and symptoms do seem to be related to cholesterol-lowering medication, it is recommended that the issue be discussed with your physician and perhaps switch to a different medication or discuss alternatives to allow you to get off of the medication altogether. Although coenzyme Q-10 is generally safe and well-tolerated, it does have the potential to thin the blood, and therefore if you are on aspirin therapy or stronger anticoagulant medication (such as Coumadin), you should consult your doctor or pharmacist before starting coenzyme Q-10.

Finally, although not technically a deficiency, some diabetics will experience symptoms in the feet that can be mistaken for plantar fasciitis that are actually due to decreased circulation. These symptoms can sometimes be helped by supplementation with alpha-lipoic acid, which is a strong anti-oxidant. For long-term use, a daily dosage of about 50 mg per day is recommended. Larger doses are sometimes recommended for short-term use, but should only be done under the supervision of a health care professional. Again, alpha-lipoic acid is a recommendation primarily for individuals who know or suspect they have diabetes which may be causing or contributing to their symptoms, and not for plantar fasciitis in and of itself.

Laser Stimulation

Use of low level or "cold" laser has become quite popular in professional pain treatment. While professional grade laser therapy equipment can be quite expensive, some therapeutic benefits can be achieved with even inexpensive laser pointers available from office supply stores (or online retailers), especially when used on a frequent basis. As with the laser suggested in the section on acupressure, I recommend using a red laser with a wavelength in the 630 nm to 635 nm range. When using a laser pointer to treat a general area of pain it's a bit different from treating acupressure points though. When used for acupressure, the laser wand was actually applied directly to the skin in order to target the specific points. For general pain relief, I recommend holding the wand a few inches away from the area of pain and then move the laser beam back and forth as if you were "painting" the entire painful area with the light.

Shoes and Arch Supports

Shoes without good arch support are likely a contributing factor in the development of plantar fasciitis and at the very least will usually slow recovery. Shoes with a high heel and that lack arch support are particularly bad as they not only allow flattening of the arches, but also tend to cause tightness in the calf muscles and Achilles tendons, which increases tension on the plantar fascia as was discussed earlier.

With that in mind, it's of course preferable to stick to low-heeled shoes that have at least some arch support in them. You can compensate for poor built-in arch support with shoe inserts or custom orthotics. For many people, over the counter shoe inserts such as gel soles or Dr. Scholl's arch supports will do a pretty good job and are pretty economical. For those with more severe arch issues though, a custom-fitted pair of orthotics may be needed. Such custom inserts can be obtained from a podiatrist, or often from chiropractors and sports medicine specialists, all of whom will typically do some sort of cast or electronic scan of the feet to determine first if you need orthotics, and second, to provide you the right orthotic for your particular needs.

Before investing hundreds of dollars in custom orthotics, I think it's worth trying the more generic ones to see if they help. If an inexpensive set of arch supports does the job, there's not really a need to spend a lot of money. If the inexpensive ones help somewhat, but don't provide quite as much relief as you hoped for, then it's a good indication that you may want to invest in custom orthotics. Be prepared that custom orthotics sometimes take a week or two to get used to and can actually increase symptoms initially. Your doctor will advise you on how to minimize symptoms during the adaptation stage, but even then, your feet may be more sore than usual, although the location of any discomfort if often different from where your plantar fasciitis symptoms are.

Magnetic Therapy

Magnetic therapy is somewhat controversial and some critics claim it is nothing more than a placebo type of treatment (the effects are imagined by people who were already expecting it to work rather than there being any real therapeutic benefit). It has been my experience that magnets do work for many people, including some who were quite skeptical initially, so I think there is more to it than a placebo effect. I do have serious doubts about the mechanism of action that many magnetic therapy devotees claim – that it works by improving circulation because the magnet pulls on the iron in the blood. I think that's pretty unlikely, and it also fails to explain why magnets help in inflammatory conditions (increasing circulation would tend to make inflammatory conditions worse). I think magnets probably work somewhat like acupuncture/acupressure, by subtly changing the flow of energy in the body. Regardless of how it works, it has been my observation that magnetic therapy is beneficial for many people.

Magnetic therapy for plantar fasciitis can take many forms, from shoe inserts to magnetic strips that can be held on, or taped to the foot, to various massagers and rollers containing magnets. For convenience of use, I suggest either insoles or a massager/roller which will provide massage effects in addition to the magnetic stimulation.

As with many other treatments, magnets can work extremely well or not at all depending on the individual. For this reason, I suggest working with either someone who sells magnets who is willing to do a demo with the products (such as with a Nikken distributor) so you can find out in advance of purchasing if they work for you, or else start with inexpensive magnetic therapy products (I suggest Lhasa-Oms.com as a resource for inexpensive magnet products).

One thing to keep in mind when using magnets is that it is possible to cause an overstimulation reaction if they are kept in place too long. In these situations, good symptomatic relief is initially achieved, but with continued use of the magnet, pain or other symptoms (tingling, numbness, etc.) may develop. This is a temporary effect and is easily remedied simply by removing the magnet for a period of time. After the side-effects of overstimulation wear off, you still can benefit from magnetic therapy, but you may want to use it for shorter periods of time, removing it for a few hours to a day whenever you reach a plateau in symptom improvement.

Energy Techniques

Hopefully you'll forgive me for going into something even weirder still than magnets, but I have found certain "energy medicine" techniques to be nearly miraculous in their effects – when they work. I was initially hesitant about including them in this book because I imagine it may damage my credibility with some readers, but since there's little harm in trying them (other than perhaps you may feel a bit silly while doing them) and potentially a big benefit, I feel I would be remiss if I did not at least offer them to you. In my 20 plus years of clinical practice, I have seen numerous cases respond to these techniques when all other treatments (of my own and of other practitioners) have failed, so while they may seem a bit odd, I encourage you to give them a try.

As with acupuncture/acupressure, there are various other ways to alter the flow of energy in the body. The first technique I will present focuses more on physical issues responsible for pain, while the second deals more with emotional issues, but I recommend that you not make any advance assumptions as to which is more appropriate for your circumstances. It is not unusual for unconscious emotional factors you're completely unaware of to trigger physical pain, so don't be too quick to rule those out even if you're the happiest, most well-adjusted person you know.

Physical Energy Balancing Method

The first technique is a very simplified version of a method I've used in my practice. The clinical version of the technique is quite involved in terms of analysis, but in my experience, the vast majority of treatment-resistant chronic pain cases, including those with plantar fasciitis, tend to have the pattern I'm going to provide you with as a major contributing factor. You will need someone to assist you in doing the procedure and that person's job will be to tap on your back as shown in the directions that follow:

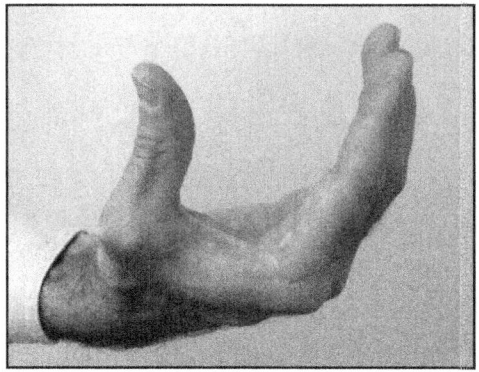

Your assistant positions his/her hand (either hand may be used) as shown so that the fingers and thumb are approximately one inch on either side of the midline of your spine.

While your assistant taps according the the instructions that follow, you will be holding one hand on the area of pain, and a finger from your other hand on your belly button as shown below. Why the belly button? Don't ask, because if you get too caught up in the weirdness of this technique, you probably won't do it and you might miss out on something that could help more than anything else you could do!

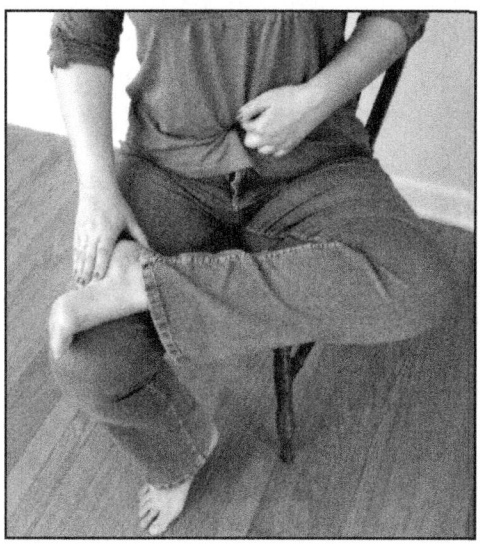

Place one of your hands on the area of pain and one finger from your other hand on your belly button.

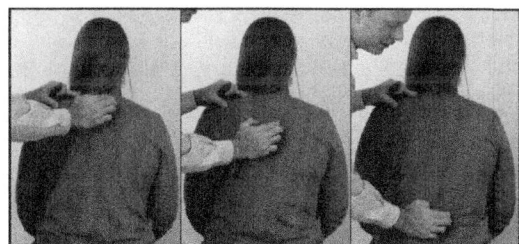

While you hold a deep breath, your assistant should begin at the top of your back and rapidly tap down the spine to your low back, moving down about half an inch with each tap. Next, as you breathe out, your assistant starts again at he top of your back and taps down the spine to your low back. Finally, as you breathe in and out rapidly (in and out about once every second), your assistant taps once more down the spine as before.

After going through the first round of holding the points and getting tapped on, re-assess the area of pain. In many cases, the location of pain will change somewhat. If so, re-position your hand to cover the new area of pain. If it requires some pressure to produce tenderness, go ahead and press on it just hard enough to produce a bit of pain, make sure to hold your belly button with your other hand, and then have your assistant repeat the procedure of tapping with the three breathing phases.

Each time through, re-assess the pain area, relocate your hand to hold any new areas of pain as before, and repeat the process. Continue repeating until you either no longer have any pain, or until you stop getting any improvement. If you don't ever get any improvement with this method after 3 or 4 tries, it's probably not going to work for you, so there's not much point in continuing. In a few cases, there is a delayed response of up to 2 days though, so if your symptoms suddenly improve in that time frame and then gradually return for no apparent reason, it may be worth trying this method again.

Be aware that after an initial relief of pain, the pain may return and even possibly get worse sometime in the next 1 to 2 days. If so, repeat the process and try the fine-tuning procedures on the video available at AskDrBest.com/pfresources.

It may take several sessions to get permanent relief of the symptoms, but as long as each session provides temporary relief, it is worthwhile to continue.

Emotional Energy Balancing – Emotional Freedom Technique (EFT)

It is not uncommon for physical pain and other symptoms to be triggered or increased by emotional factors. There are many methods for handling negative emotional states, but one of the simplest methods I've found that is well-suited to self-treatment is called Emotional Freedom Technique, or EFT for short.

Emotional Freedom Technique is most often used as a means of handling negative emotions and as a means of habit control, but it can be very helpful in dealing with pain as well. EFT combines acupressure with verbal affirmations to change energy flow through the body that is related to emotions (even ones you're not consciously aware of). I will summarize the basic procedure here and most people will do quite well just using the basics, but you can also download a free full-length manual on this method, as well as get information on seminars and advanced instruction by going to www.EFTuniverse.com.

As I said, Emotional Freedom Technique uses acupressure stimulation along with verbal affirmations to change the "emotional charge" or intensity of a physical pain, craving, habit, phobia, or traumatic event. The starting point of the procedure is to identify whatever it is you want to change, and then verbalize it in the form of a self-accepting affirmation while tapping a series of points.

For example, let's say you are experiencing plantar fasciitis symptoms. For the purposes of doing Emotional Freedom Technique, you will always use the structure of "Even though I [insert undesirable symptom, behavior, or emotion here], I deeply and completely accept myself." So, using the example of plantar fasciitis, you would say, "Even though I am having plantar fasciitis, I deeply and completely accept myself." Alternately in this case, you might say something like, "Even though I am having pain in my foot, I deeply and completely accept myself."

In the case of pain and other symptoms, you may be able to associate a certain emotional event or stressful situation to the onset or increase of the symptoms. In fact, sometimes simply noticing the words we use can clue us in on emotional issues that may be triggering physical symptoms.

Even though most cases of plantar fasciitis are related to physical problems in the foot, you might be surprised at how much of a role emotional issues can play and sometimes you may even find a clue in things you find yourself saying. For instance, if you feel stuck in a given situation and say things like how you wish you could just "move forward" or "take the necessary steps" to deal with the situation, you may very well experience increased physical pain in your foot (the physical manifestation of not being able to move forward or take steps). This may all sound kind of like "woo-woo" psychobabble, but you might be surprised at how much of an issue it can be with chronic physical pain.

Diminishing the "charge" of underlying emotional issues can bring a surprising amount of pain relief in some cases. Although other techniques for using affirmations may recommend phrasing your affirmations in terms of the way you want things to be (such as, "I feel healthy and pain-free!"), this in not how they are used with Emotional Freedom Technique. So, as another example, let's say that you recognize an emotional issue such as frustration with not being able to move forward with something may be participating in your physical symptoms. You could use the affirmation, "Even though I haven't been able to move forward, I deeply and completely accept myself."

Whatever the affirmation for your specific issue, you repeat it out loud as you tap a series of acupressure points. The sequence and location of the points is shown below. For each point, you'll tap it 7 or 8 times with a finger tip as you repeat the affirmation out loud. Tap the points in the number sequence shown, starting at point 1 above the eye and working through to point 13 (if you download the full manual from the Emotional Freedom Technique website, you'll see that I have added one finger point – this point is optional and I have included it only because it is easier to just do all of the fingers than try to remember which one you don't need to do).

It usually does not matter whether you do points on the left or right side of the body, but I find it usually works better to stick to one side, rather than doing some points on the left and some on the right. You may find that tapping the points on the side of pain works the best.

Points for Emotional Freedom Technique:

(The points are illustrated on the pictures that follow.)

1. Over Eye

2. Outside Corner of Eye

3. Under Eye

4. Between Nose and Upper Lip

5. Between Lower Lip and Chin

6. Just Below Where Collar Bone Joins Breastbone

7. Center of Arm Pit

8. Outer Edge of Base of Thumb Nail

9. Outer Edge (Thumb Side) of Base of Index Finger Nail

10. Outer Edge (Thumb Side) of Base of Middle Finger Nail

11. Outer Edge (Thumb Side) of Base of Ring Finger Nail

12. Outer Edge (Thumb Side) of Base of Little ("Pinky") Finger Nail

13. "Karate Chop" Point On Outer Edge of Hand Midway Between Little Finger and Wrist

Plantar Fasciitis Exercises and Home Treatment • 39

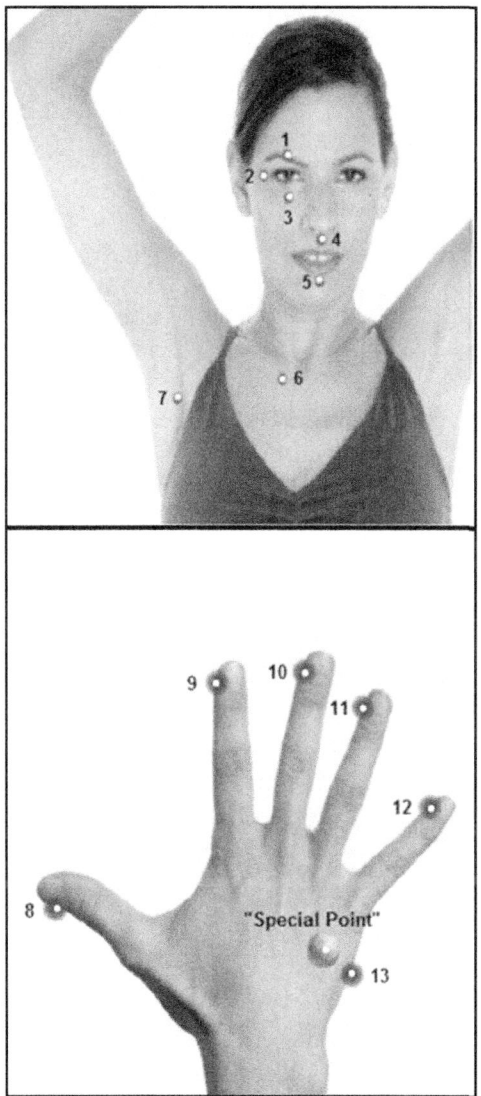

After you have tapped on the series of points while repeating the affirmation ("Even though I [insert undesirable symptom, behavior, or emotion here], I deeply and completely accept myself."), the next step is to activate various brain centers while tapping on what I'll call the "special point" point on the back of the hand, on a line directly between the ring finger and little finger, midway between the base of the fingers and the wrist (as shown on the hand image in the picture above).

As you tap on the "special point", you'll go through a series of steps as follows:

1. Open your eyes.

2. Close your eyes.

3. Open your eyes and, without moving your head, look down and left with your eyes.

4. Open your eyes and, without moving your head, look down and right with your eyes.

5. Circle ("roll") your eyes clockwise.

6. Circle ("roll") your eyes counter-clockwise.

7. Hum a tune for a few seconds (any familiar tune will work, such as the "Happy Birthday" song).

8. Count out loud from one to five ("one, two, three, four, five").

9. Hum a tune again for a few seconds.

Once you have completed these procedures while tapping the "special point", there's one more step. Once again, you will tap 7 or 8 times on each of the 13 points done in the initial step, this time while repeating just the phrase that describes the undesirable symptom, habit, behavior, or emotion. For example, if your affirmation in the first step of the procedure was, "Even though I have foot pain, I deeply and completely accept myself.", this time through you will repeat just the phrase, "foot pain" while you tap the points.

After one time through the entire procedure, most people will have significant improvement in the symptoms, habit, behavior, or emotion they wish to change. If there is no improvement, you may want to think about underlying issues that are related to the problem you wish to address. For example, if your pain started shortly after a major fight with your wife about your finances, you might switch from a symptom-focused affirmation like "Even though I have foot pain…" to "Even though I disagree with my wife about our finances…".

If there is some, but not 100% improvement, the procedure can be repeated with a variation in the affirmation used in the initial step and the phrase used in the final step. For repeats of the procedure, there is an acknowledgment of the prior issue being somewhat improved.

For example, if the first time through the procedure your affirmation was, "Even though I have sciatica, I deeply and completely accept myself.", your affirmation for the first step each time you repeat the procedure will be, "Even though I *still have some remaining foot pain*, I deeply and completely accept myself.". And for the final step of the procedure for the repeats, the phrase would change from "foot pain" to "remaining foot pain". Otherwise, the procedure for repeats is the same as when you do it the first time for a given issue.

In some cases, you may need to get more specific with your affirmation to help with the problem you are experiencing. For instance, if you are having problems with left heel pain, it may be more effective to say, "Even though I have pain in my left heel…" than to say "Even though I have foot pain…". The more specific you can be and the more you can deal with any possible emotional triggers for your pain, the more effective EFT will be.

Visit AskDrBest.com/pfresources for video instructions for performing EFT.

Chapter 3: Professional Treatment

While this book is mainly intended to provide self treatment solutions for plantar fasciitis, there are times when professional treatment may be needed and/or may speed up the recovery process.

Prescription Medication

Although still a very popular treatment, medication is minimally helpful at best in most cases of plantar fasciitis. The medications prescribed tend to be anti-inflammatory drugs of some sort. As was discussed in the first chapter, although plantar fasciitis was once thought to be primarily an inflammatory process, recent studies have found that in most cases, there is little inflammation present, and the condition is actually a degenerative process. Because of this, it's not really surprising that anti-inflammatory drugs have little effect. Most anti-inflammatory medications have some pain-suppressing effects, so they may help a little bit, but for most people with plantar fasciitis they really don't do very much.

Strong pain medications will suppress the symptoms, but they do nothing to actually help resolve the problem and symptoms return as soon as the medication wears off. Since pain medications will often dull the mind and make it difficult to work and maintain focus, they really are not a good long-term solution in most cases.

Physical Therapy

Physical therapy is a rather broad field of health care and can include a variety of different treatment methods. With regards specifically to plantar fasciitis, there's a handful of techniques that are commonly employed.

Ultrasound Therapy

Ultrasound therapy uses high-frequency sound waves to produce a subtle vibration in the tissues, resulting in deep heat that enhances circulation and relaxes contracted soft tissues. It can be very effective in providing temporary relief from symptoms associated with plantar fasciitis and/or heel spurs. With repeated sessions, it may provide enough improvement to produce lasting symptom relief. Ultrasound can be applied by itself or in combination with analgesic gels/lotions which the ultrasonic waves may help to penetrate the tissue more deeply (in which case, the therapy is called phonophoresis).

Iontophoresis

Iontophoresis is a technique that, like phonophoresis, drives analgesic medications faster and deeper into the tissue than would occur just by normal absorption. Where phonophoresis uses sound waves, iontophoresis uses electric current, which itself has some potential pain relief benefits. The effects of iontophoresis are generally temporary, but it can ease symptoms sufficiently to allow exercises and other treatments to be performed more comfortably.

Massage Therapy

Massage has been discussed as a self-treatment measure, but of course professional massage treatment is also available. Massage is offered in many physical therapy clinics as well as through independent licensed massage therapists. Deep tissue techniques are usually the most effective for plantar fasciitis, and it is often helpful to have work done not only in the foot, but also in the legs and back, as there is interdependence of the musculoskeletal structures throughout the body.

Taping

Some physical therapists will employ specialized taping techniques to provide support to the foot and ankle with the intention of promoting healing. Properly done taping can be quite effective as a short-term treatment for plantar fasciitis and not only provides symptom relief, but can assist in healing by means of reducing mechanical stress on the damaged tissue. You may find "do-it-yourself" guides to taping in books and online, but unless you have experience with taping, it's best to work with a professional at least at first so that you know how to apply the tape properly. Books and even video instructions don't do a very good job of teaching you how tightly the tape should be applied, so some hands-on instruction is highly recommended before you attempt to do your own taping.

Extracorporeal Shock Wave Therapy

Extracorporeal shock wave therapy (ESWT) is a relatively new and somewhat controversial treatment for plantar fasciitis. Although it is non-surgical therapy, it tends to be performed more by medical doctors than by physical therapists. This treatment was originally developed for non-surgical removal of kidney stones. It works by firing a powerful sound wave pulse into the tissue.

In the case of plantar fasciitis, ESWT is thought to work by producing micro-trauma in the degenerating tissue which triggers the body's inflammatory and healing mechanisms. There are high energy and low energy shock wave treatments that may be used. The low energy systems are somewhat more popular due to the fact that the treatments (usually done as a series of three sessions) are usually not painful and can be done without anesthesia. The high energy form of the treatment usually requires only one session, but it can be quite painful and usually requires either regional or general anesthesia. Research on the effectiveness of ESWT has shown mixed results, so the usefulness of this form of treatment is still in debate.

Chiropractic / Osteopathic Manipulation

Although chiropractic and osteopathic manipulation is more commonly associated with treatments delivered to the spine of the back and neck, manipulation can be used on extra-spinal joints (meaning joints outside of the spine) as well. In the case of plantar fasciitis, chiropractors/osteopaths trained in extra-spinal analysis and manipulation techniques will evaluate and correct misalignments or faulty mobility patterns in the foot, ankle, and perhaps joints further up in the skeleton as well, such as the sacroiliac joints and lumbar spinal joints. By correcting joint alignment and mobility of these areas, mechanical stresses on the plantar fascia can be reduced, and healing can be facilitated. *Note – not all practitioners who do manipulation are trained in extra-spinal techniques, so be sure to ask about this specifically before setting an appointment.

Acupuncture

As you might expect given the section on self-treatment with acupressure, I recommend acupuncture as a professional treatment option. Acupuncture needles are extremely thin and usually don't produce the type of pain that may be experienced with things like injections or blood draws, so most people tolerate them quite well. Even so, although some acupuncturists only use needles, many also offer the options of acupressure or laser or electrical acupuncture for those who may be "needle-phobic".

Regardless of what is used to stimulate the points, a skilled acupuncturist will analyze your energy balance through various techniques and thereby can provide a customized treatment that may be much more effective than the general acupressure recommendations found in this book.

Injections

There are two main types of injections used in the treatment of plantar fasciitis. The most common type is the injection of cortisone or some other type of corticosteroid, the primary purpose of which is to reduce inflammation. Again, since most cases of plantar fasciitis are not caused by inflammation, this treatment is usually not dramatically effective, but old habits die hard in health care and steroid injections remain a fairly popular treatment. Steroid injections can be very effective in some cases, leading to speculation that there are indeed some situations where inflammation plays a role, or possibly that the act of simply inserting the injection needle might have a therapeutic effect of some kind, such as through the energy balancing of acupuncture, or through the mechanisms of stimulating inflammation and tissue healing (such as those theorized for extracorporeal shock wave therapy and the second type of injections we're about to discuss).

The second type of injection used to treat plantar fasciitis is called prolotherapy and it involves injecting irritating substances into areas of soft tissue damage/degeneration with the intention of provoking an inflammatory response. While on the surface, that may sound counter-intuitive as a treatment, there is evidence that by provoking the inflammatory response, the healing processes of the body are essentially re-started. In essence, the concept of prolotherapy is that it stimulates the body to make a new attempt at healing an area that may not have healed properly initially. However it works, prolotherapy has been beneficial for many people with chronic pain syndromes. It certainly is not 100% effective, but I believe it merits consideration in cases that have been resistant to other types of treatment.

Custom Fitted Orthotics

Orthotics were discussed previously, but I wanted to briefly discuss custom-fitted orthotics in more detail. While there are stores where you can purchase custom orthotics outside of a clinical setting, the majority are actually prescribed items provided by podiatrists and chiropractors. There are many different brands of custom orthotics and a variety of ways that are used to analyze the feet to arrive at the specific customizations. Regardless of brand and analysis method, there are two main types of professionally prescribed orthotics that are commonly seen – rigid and semi-flexible.

While it is my opinion that there is no inherently superior system of analysis for prescribing orthotics, nor a superior brand, I do strongly favor semi-flexible orthotics over the rigid type, especially for anyone who spends a lot of time on their feet and/or who engages in running or other athletic activities. Rigid orthotics are basically hard pieces of plastic with no padding or shock absorbing material. While they will provide extremely stable arch support, most people I've seen who have tried them could not tolerate wearing them all day and they were especially problematic for anyone who tried to run with them in their shoes. By contrast, most semi-flexible orthotics do have shock-absorbing materials built into them and they move somewhat with the foot through the gait cycle. Semi-flexible orthotics can sometimes cause increased foot soreness during the initial adjustment phase, but after that it has been my experience that most people are very pleased with them.

Rest

Although it's not as common of a recommendation as it once was, rest (sometimes total bed rest without putting any pressure on the feet at all for days, weeks, or even months) is still occasionally recommended in the treatment of plantar fasciitis. While there may be some exceptions in extreme cases of foot trauma where short-term rest is appropriate, it generally is not a good strategy for recovering from plantar fasciitis. Although symptoms do usually improve during a prolonged period of rest, plantar fasciitis will usually rapidly return as soon as weight bearing on the feet is resumed – often worse than before the resting regimen was implemented. While extreme exertion such as distance running, or high impact activities like jumping may need to be curtailed temporarily in the initial stages of treatment, prolonged rest without putting any weight on the feet usually causes more harm than good.

Night Bracing

Night bracing of the ankle in the position doctors call "dorsiflexion" in which the top of the foot is stretched towards the front of the shin can be an effective treatment for plantar fasciitis. Such bracing provides what is essentially a prolonged calf stretch. Like any other method of calf stretching, the intention is to reduce backward and upward tension on the heel bone that in turn increases tension on the plantar fascia. While most people will get satisfactory results from periodic stretching sessions, night bracing can speed up recovery in those people who are poorly compliant with the recommended stretching regimens and/or who have unusually tight calf muscles and Achilles tendons.

Surgery

Finally we come to surgery, and as it is the last treatment to be discussed in this book, in my opinion it should be the very last treatment option considered for plantar fasciitis. In rare cases, plantar fasciitis may be so treatment resistant that all non-surgical options will fail to provide satisfactory results. Unfortunately, even surgery may be ineffective in such cases, but if all other treatments have been exhausted, surgery may be warranted.

There are a couple of different surgical procedures that can be done. One involves lengthening the calf muscles to reduce tension on the Achilles tendon and its attachment on the heel bone. As with calf stretching, the goal here is to reduce tension on the plantar fascia.

The other procedure is an incision part way through the plantar fascia itself, with the goal of allowing it to lengthen slightly. This procedure may be combined with the removal of a heel spur if present.

Neither of these procedures is a sure thing, and even with initial success, post-surgical scar tissue can negate the beneficial effects over time. Even the Academy of Orthopedic Surgeons (a group that overall tends to have a relatively positive view of surgery) has stated that plantar fasciitis surgery should only be considered "after 12 months of aggressive nonsurgical treatment". So, just in case you didn't get the point – don't be in a rush to do surgery as it usually responds well to non-surgical treatment and surgical results can be very disappointing.

In Conclusion

Although plantar fasciitis can be a frustrating condition to deal with, the vast majority of cases do get better with time and usually do not require surgical intervention. The home treatment methods discussed in this book when applied as directed will accelerate recovery in most cases and will often provide substantial relief or even elimination of symptoms within a few days to a few weeks. Resistant cases may take longer, but regardless of recovery time, it should be remembered that for many people the underlying causes for developing plantar fasciitis in the first place are still things they are exposed to in their day to day lives. For this reason, investing a few minutes each day in performing the exercises and other treatments (whichever ones you found most helpful) for preventive purposes will help you avoid a potential return of symptoms.

Review and Connect

I hope you have found this book helpful and if so, I ask that you consider posting a review on your favorite book retailer's website and/or any book review sites you enjoy.

For additional information, and/or if you have questions or comments regarding this book, I may be contacted via:

My website: http://www.AskDrBest.com/pfresources

My Facebook page: https://www.facebook.com/AskDrBest

Printed in Great Britain
by Amazon

26768220R00031